I0447281

Printed May 2012
Cover Design By Greg Ryan
Editing by Greg Ryan
ISBN 978-1475230147

Trainer Dude 100

Things I Did Not Learn In a Classroom!

About the Author

At age 46, a Greg a native of St. Joseph Michigan has amassed a striking list of credentials. What began at age sixteen, Greg over a span of thirty years has accomplish everything one could imagine in the health and fitness industry; specifically the personal training profession.

In 1990 he moved to Los Angeles California, where his knowledge enthusiasm and skill attracted the attention of fitness guru Kathy Smith. During this time Greg ran one of the largest personal training businesses in LA. Attracting numerous high profile movies stars. Greg built a reputation for exercise and behavior change and in the fall of 1992 appeared on the Today Show and Good Morning America.

Greg's produced his own television segment on FOX TV in the mid nineties while attending Physical Therapy school. In 1997 Greg relocated to Louisville Kentucky were he operated an ever so growing private clinic specializing in obesity, diabetes and weight loss programs.

In the fall of 2004 Greg authored and published his first of a total of twenty-four books to-dated on fitness, personal training, body building, steroids and disease.

As it relates to RICH TRAINER POOR TRAINER, over the last thirty years Greg has acquired nearly one hundred thousand hours of paid personal training sessions and designed and help build a dozen or more training facilities. In that time he has learned some of the best kept secrets to being successful as a fitness trainer in both, good and bad economic times.

Why should you read this book?

Every personal trainer who has NOT made a million dollars in the fitness business needs to read the RICH TRAINER, POOR TRAINER series, or at the very least this book, TRAINER DUDE 100.   Any one in the fitness industry should read it, for that matter.

Who is Greg Ryan?

Well, there was a time growing up that I wasn't sure. Not a confident dude, nor did I have the slightest idea of the direction my life would take. Farm boy by trade with a discipline only instilled by the day to day work in the trenches; I guess, God saw something I didn't. What in the world could he do with an introverted, unmotivated medium educated boy from a small town in Michigan?

Well, fitness found me and personally changed it all; probably more like he unlocked the key to the real guy inside; fitness was just the vehicle to better things.

How did it all happen?

The beginning was just a blur, it was challenging just to ride the wave. First the opportunity to compete as a bodybuilder was completely different than anything I had done or had the personality for. Follow that up with finding myself in a well respected leadership role of coaching others on fitness was, at the time almost laughable; besides the fact of making money at it. How did I get into fitness training, "*Accidental Coincidences,*" I say? Fitness found me and I found a career. Four lines on a piece of paper and three decades later, here I am.

Maybe I was just at the right place at the right time in my life, I don't know? Maybe it was accidentally walking through the wrong door at college, where I met two of what ended up being the greatest friends and support I could ever have? Or maybe it was truly those four lines I wrote on that scrap paper as a teenager that read,

"Only by the Grace of God in America

could one get paid, be prosperous and live their dream,

by teaching people to strive for healthy lives through exercise.

LORD, let that be me."

Looking back, maybe it was just me being naive enough to believe those words that put me in the car that day? Oh that day, I remember it well, August 17, 1989. With five hundreds dollars to my name, no job or direction holding just a hope in my heart and a dream in my mind, I left the world only as I knew it in search of a what, I was not sure? What I am sure of is, there are no coincidences in life, no accidental circumstances that just happen to find you. We all have our place in this life to touch just the right person at the most appropriate time. How did it all happen, I'm not sure how, but I do know why?

Why have I stayed?

I have stayed, because of how it all happened. I have stayed in the fitness business because of my promise I made to myself and those that I am yet to have met. The day I left for California I decided that fitness training was my calling; the very thing that I was born to do. It had changed my life, saved it more less, and now through me

I must help change another. I have stayed thirty years due to that promise and because I have yet to meet the one for the very reason it has all started in the first place.

What is RICH- TRAINER- POOR TRAINER?

My life I guess you could say. This book series is an accumulation of my experiences, trials, tribulations, mistakes and triumphs that I would not change for all the money in the world. RICH TRAINER -POOR TRAINER is to me one of the only and most important ways I could ever give back to the industry what it as given me; knowledge, wisdom, gratification, courage, belief and even peace. What is RICH TRAINER- POOR TRAINER, priceless in my opinion? And it is my prayer that if you are serious about the fitness training profession, you too will decide to read it.

From the Author

I am all for institutional education. In this business it's a must, but only as a foundation not a pass. While I am glad I completed my requirements as far as school goes, my true education came from OJT not a PHD. OJT or *"On the Job Training,"* is where you find the real tests, the real answers and the real world.

Today, fitness trainers make the vital mistake of hiding behind their accomplishments in the classroom, thinking that's all there is too it and they will become successful. News flash, not even close to the truth! Success is not in the x's and o's of a chart, but in the people themselves.

Trainer Dude 100 is a collection of things that I have observed and learned from the *"Real"* world through sweat equity, time, and my very own mistakes. This may be the most important book of the series, so I advise you to listen and take heed to every statement put forth in this book. **It WILL be the difference between you being *Rich* or *Poor* in the fitness training business.**

Content

The "X" Factor- *The Gift*

Business 101- *Sold Out*

Ethics 101- *The Right Thing*

Psychology 101- *Competitive to Creative*

Common Sense 101- *The Price of Ignorance*

People 101- *The "Art" of People Training*

Leadership 101-*Silence Speaks Volumes*

Marking 101 *Leveraging Your Brand*

Nutrition 101- *The Big Picture*

Gym Owners/Fitness Directors -*Less is More*

Bonus Material

Trainer Dude 101- *The "Art" of Training*

Do not make your profession in the fitness world complicated, it's not. Don't think that you have arrived at any point in your career, because that will be the beginning of the end for you. Do however, compete only with yourself, fuel the creativity inside; never fall prey to small minded thinking on the outside and love people for who they are not what you want them to become.

Greg Ryan

Introduction

There is no better education than hands on experience. There are no substitutes for it either. Neither a piece of paper nor a person can just give it too you. You earn it, by getting up in the morning, following your dreams and striving toward a purpose. More times than not, true learning comes not in comforting times but, challenging ones.

The fitness training business is a learning experience daily. One day you may learn something about a client, another time it could be about the profession itself; then there are those times you learn hard lessons about yourself. But, every situation is archived into your own little library of memories to be avoided or built upon at later times in your life.

The adventurous part of the fitness training business is you will never learn everything. Some think they have, but in the end are swallowed up by their own pride. Fitness training as a business takes mental flexibility and fortitude. Sure there are medical guidelines to follow, but in the end it's about people and fore sight, not a charts, graphs or immediate gratification.

Just surviving as a fitness trainer is challenging enough, but being successful year after year takes something special, and it takes working smart every single day.

My goal with in these pages is to give you a little taste of what I have learned through my very own day to day experiences over the past thirty years. Conducting close to one hundred thousand hours of fitness training sessions, you can't help but learn a few valuable things about people's behaviors and needs, the business itself and what makes you tick as well.

The statements or rules are in no order of importance based on their numbers, however, I guess you could say, "They ALL are important in there own application."

Be careful as you read these hundred or so little quotes and explanations. There are a lot of important things to learn between the lines. However, they are only as good as your implementation into your own life, career and business.

The "X" Factor
"The Gift"

Why is it that some people become successful and others do not? You can take two people who do the exact same thing in a business and have two totally different results. Is one person just luckier than the other? Or do they just know and have something most do not?

A RICH fitness trainer and a POOR one are separated by two things; how they think and how they use what God has given them. Sounds simply, but if that were the case, why are there not more successful fitness trainers or coaches?

"How have you been able to stay in the business of personal training, let alone be very successful at it?"

You have got to have something extra, know and care for people, use common sense and set up the right business template. RICH trainers have a quality that can not be taught, it is what I call the, **"X" Factor.** In other words, you need to be the Simon Cowell of fitness.

Here are a few things I learned about the importance of the "X" factor.

1. **Find your "Gift," harness it and ride the wave for the rest of your life.**

Each person has something they are good at. Discover what it is and apply daily.

2. **Be careful how you think, small town thinking will cost you dreams and cash.**

Believe in bigger things, not what others tell you to do.

3. **Your income is in direct relation to your self-worth.**

If you believe you can or can't the outcome will be the same.

4. **Simplicity goes a long way, and makes you more money with less effort in the end.**

Don't complicate your career, people or your training methods, keep it real and simple.

5. **Nurture Creativity and snuff out Competitiveness.**
Constantly be imaginative and flexible and avoid competing with others. Focus on a better you.

6. Love it or Leave it!

No matter the money or the prestige if you resent getting out of bed for work, don't. Love your job or leave it!

7. Love yourself, respect your profession.

Care deeply for your wellbeing without ego; never think you are above reproach.

8. Give to Get

Before you can receive anything you have to be willing to give it away; time, generosity, money, energy.

9. It's not about the money.

If you are a fitness trainer just to make money you will NEVER be successful.

10. There are no options!

When times get tough, you remember there are no options, but to move forward.

It's not about you, when it comes to the success of your <u>clients.</u> *It's IS all about you* when it comes to the success of your <u>business.</u>

Greg Ryan

Business 101
"Sold Out"

Personal or Fitness Training is a *"Business."* Attitudes, Philosophies, Principles, Structure, Policies and Goals all must be a part of the developmental planning of that business. You are either sold out too your career or you're not, but, that's just the start. Long term, you are only as good as those you surround yourself with, and how well you implement your business principles. Here are a few things pertaining to the business aspect of training I have learned,

11. *"Lifers"* **make more money than, *"Part Timers."***

Have a *"Sold Out,"* attitude about your career and business from the beginning. And yes, it is a business!!

12. **Freedom comes with a price, but when you get it, it's priceless.**

Eventually, the only way to prosperity is to work for your self.

13. **Be *"Great"* at little rather than mediocre with a lot.**

Find a niche and be good at it. Don't complicate or dilute for the sake of ego.

14. Slave to the Lender- Avoid Bad Debt!

Avoid bad debt at all cost. Burdens cost money and squelches creativity.

15. Embrace "OJT," On the Job Training and nurture PHD or Education.

Classroom education is a must, but experience is the real teacher.

16. Develop *"Gate Keepers"* to protect your business interests.

Surround your business quality business minded people.

17. Do not get above your business.

Humility is the key to prosperity; ego is the brother of poverty.

18. Pillow talk is a disease of the mind and heart and your business will die of a slow hidden death.

Avoid personal relationships with employees, clients or business associates.

19. Business success is not based on numbers, it's gauged by longevity.

Concentrate on keeping your clients more than trying to get new ones; energy and money better spent.

20. Accountability is more important than compromise.

Establishing boundaries, enforcing business policies and holding people to their goals is more rewarding and cash generating in the end than negotiating your principles.

Do the right thing, even if it's not popular.

Trainer Ethics 101
"Doing the Right Thing"

How you conduct your fitness training career is your business. But, understand that life will have its say, sooner or later. The success of your business is up to you, not your clients; how you go about getting it may be more important than the wealth, status or experience that you want to acquire.

Ethics by definition are moral principles you have inside you. Your actions at their core are determined by such morals. And life will either reward you for them or turn on you because of them. Your ethical beliefs affect yourself, others and your profession as a whole, remember that.

Each day you will have to decide; follow what is right, even when it may not be popular, or compromise everything for the sake of the moment or circumstances. We live and die by our daily decisions. Here are some ethical standards to live by,

21. Let your actions speak so loud that when you talk they can not hear you.

Make sure your actions align with what you believe in and how you are acting.

22. If it's not popular with others in your profession, chances are it's the right thing to do.

Do the right thing even if it's not popular or the norm of those trainers around you.

23. The truth about Karma, it's real.

Do not under cut, back stab or talk about another trainer or fitness profession, it will only make you and the profession look and feel bad.

24. Say what you mean, and mean what you say.

Political Correctness in the fitness business is an enabler.

25. One bad apple spoils the bunch.

Don't cast a bad light on an already disrespected profession by, acting in an unethical way.

26. Avoid being a "Wolf Spider" at all costs.

Wolf spiders eat their own. Do not talk about other trainers or bad mouth them to others. It will only come back to bite you.

27. Dishonesty brings strife and poverty to your heart and business.

No matter what, tell your clients the truth, you own them at least that. Your increase in income will show.

Free Your Mind and the Rest Will Follow!

Psychology 101
Free Your Mind

Psychology is a vital part of the process within your self. Competition comes not from the world as much as it does from with in.

We control our lives and career by our thoughts and beliefs. Creativity and Gratitude are the cornerstones to success both emotionally and financially. Here are a few tips to think about when managing your own mind and fitness career.

28. A busy mind is the center of an unaccomplished career.

Practice quiet or meditation time; clients and money will then knock at your door.

29. Think creatively, and avoid competing.

Imagination attracts money, while competitive thinking or being concerned about another repels it.

30. You receive what you believe you are worth.

Your income is in direct relationship to how much confidence you have in your abilities.

31. You do not have because you do not ask.

Don't be afraid to ask for business.

32. The minds eye does NOT know right from wrong.

Never underestimate the power of visualizing your business, future and income.

33. If you want money, be grateful for what you have first.

Gratitude is the key to open the door too the bank vault.

34. Your "Will" controls your pocket book.

Believe it or not, you can "Will," things into existence, if you are strong enough to do the emotional work.

35. Free your mind and the rest will follow.

Your mind is your biggest competitor, not life, other trainers or the economy. Free it up and watch what happens.

Common Sense 101
The Price of Ignorance

Common sense is not learned or given as a gift; you either possess it, or you don't. Practicing good judgment in your business is as important as exercising is to losing weight.

When dealing with people, your business or the profession incorporating a common sense approach to things is best. It's important to understand; it will take you twice as long and much more energy and money to succeed with out it; assuming that you do. Here are a few common sense things I have learned about fitness training,

36. Ignorance is the absence of common sense.

With out having a common sense approach to your business, you will most likely not see failure coming.

37. Ego is a money stealer, humility is a money giver.

Your Ego will cost you more money than anything else in your career.

38. Story tell for money

If people can relate to a story then you got them emotionally connected. Common sense is sometimes in the form of a story.

39. Common sense may cost you a few cents

Practicing good judgment in your business may cost you a penny in the beginning but in the end will allow you to have more cents.

40. Lack of Common sense sank the Titanic

If you think you are above reproach or your business is better than the rest your business (ship) is already sinking; and only a matter of time.

People 101

Success is measured in relationships not numbers. People are attracted to caring more than knowing. EQ reaches hearts more than IQ.

Every person is different, so your approach must be. Master the *"Art"* of People and the cash will be there for the taking. Here are some people skills and thoughts,

41. Relationships equal retention

Invest in developing professional relationships with clients and the financial payoff will be long term.

42. EQ is more important and lucrative than IQ.

Motivating people is more emotional than intellectual. Learn people and the x's and o's are easy.

43. One size does not fit all.

One type of exercise approach does not work for everyone. You have to address personality types to succeed.

EQ is more lucrative than IQ.

44. Give responsibility and expect accountability.

People feel better about themselves when accomplishing things or assignments; however, sometimes they need to be made to do so.

45. Train based on Personality not

Two types of personalities need two different approaches.

46. Assumptions are expensive.

Do not assume about peoples income, likeness of you, buying power or commitment level.

47. Give people what they NEED, not what they want.

Hold people accountable to their goals, they WANT that.

48. People don't expect you to know everything, but they do expect honesty.

Admit you may not know an answer, by being honest ALL the time.

Let your actions speak so loudly that when you speak they can not hear you!

Leadership 101
Lead with Silence

Being a good Leader requires guts, a spine and faith. In the fitness business you are paid to lead, no matter what. Holding an adult in this world accountable for their actions goes against the grain, and at times is not politically correct, so what. Leaders are lonely at the top by nature. Lead or follow that's your choice. Here are few leadership things to ponder,

49. No guts no glory.

Leadership requires confidence, confidence makes money.

50. Empty words are like getting free advice and then they send you the bill.

Don't be a hypocrite. Through your actions, make your words have weight behind them.

51. Honesty and transparency builds cash bridges.

If you don't know an answer, say you don't, and find it out. People know when you are BS them.

52. Leading sometimes means NOT leading.

Leaders learn to say no when need be. If you are a yes person, you are a poor one too.

53. Lead by sometimes doing the opposite.

Stick with YOUR plan even if it means sometimes going against the grain of your peers.

54. Lead by empowering, not degrading.

Inspiration with accountability and love is always more profitable than with degradation and fear.

Marketing 101
Leveraging you Brand

Marketing and Branding is a necessity in the fitness training business. Work smart or waste cash, not easy to predetermine. The art is in the leveraging. The power is in your Brand. Like a lot of things, it's not rocket science, but it does require discipline, dedication and perseverance.

The key is to not forget the best way of building relationships, at the same time not be left behind in today's social media world and technology. Here are a few tips I've learned,

55. Either you stand for something or you fall for anything.

Making a name means being the same person all the time. Decide your identity and never deviate.

56. Never deface your logo.

Never add too your logo, once out there; it lessens the power of your brand; by confusing the market.

Branding says nothing with out Leverage

57. Branding is about consistency, not hard selling.

When creating a name for yourself, focus on being consistent with something more than in your face selling.

58. Without trust, marketing means nothing.

No matter how you market your brand, you have to consistently build trust between you and your clients.

59. Personal and Social go together in today's world.

You will not succeed as a fitness trainer today with out marketing with social media and building personal face to face relationships.

60. Good marketers build a following through education not sales promotions.

Building a group of followers today is about consistently educating, not selling them.

K.I.S.S.

Keep it simple!

Nutrition 101
Big Picture

Dealing with food is an "Attitude," as much as it is counting calories; maybe even more so. You always have to look at food from

Keeping the big picture in mind, does not mean you have to be a dietician. You can educate and encourage while at the same time, not confuse or complicate. A fitness trainer's purpose is more in the follow through rather than the food itself. Leave the hard stuff to someone else. Here are some things to chew on when implementing nutrition advice in your business,

70. Chose your battles carefully.

You are not a dietician, don't claim to be.

71. Food and fitness is more about accountability than calorie counting.

A trainer's job is more of encouraging awareness of eating habits than solving the x's and o's.

72. Playing psychologist and therapist is part of the job.

Changing eating habits is about discovering emotional attachments to food, and changing them.

73. Emotional accountability is physically harder than any exercise responsibility.
Holding people accountability to good eating habits at home takes emotion confidence, more so than making then run.

74. Push too hard, deprivation steps in, encourage to little, perseverance gives in.

Changing ones food habits is a long process; too many boundaries people rebel, not enough guidelines they lose hope and confidence.

75. Play the percentages.

Do not get too hung up on micro managing, help your clients learn the percentage of types of foods, not always a calorie issue.

Gym Owner - Fitness Director 101
Motivate for More Money

The goal, increase cash flow and decrease turn over. Owners and Directors seek fairness and balance with fitness trainers. Here are a few things to think about in managing this part of your business,

76. Complacency breeds poverty

Gym owners, managers or directors should never lose touch with their staff by hiding in their office.

77. Cultivate relationships with honesty

Map out in writing all your businesses guidelines and policies. Make sure they understand in writing what is expected of them.

78. Creativity spawns cash flow.

Be open and get your trainers involved in creating incentive programs for themselves. Who said you have to do the industry norm?

Decrease turn over- Increase Cash Flow

79. Consistency Pays

What ever trainer policy you implement, do it consistently will ALL trainers. Favors undermine your authority.

80. CYA

Cover your butt. Require liability insurance always. At the very least, it builds respect between you and the trainer.

81. Clothing optional

Depending on your trainer policy, it's always best to have a dress code.

82. Cash flow by committee

Create a manager on duty program; one person in charge of the floor for a period of time. Confidence creates cash.

83. Confine and Conquer

Confine all drama and disputes to each individual. Conquer it before it gets out of control, and you lose control.

The money is in the "Art!"

Bonus Material

The "Art" of Fitness Training 101

Fitness Training is an *"Art"* as much as it is a profession. If you are fortunate to get results consistently, you may survive. After thirty years I have been blessed to have built a small fortune because I have never forgotten the little things during a client training session that makes all the world of difference in their success and mine in the end.

It's not rocket science, but you have to, even for a session take your mind off yourself and put yourself in the shoes of the person. Here are a few training session tips that have made me a million that you should ALWAYS do,

84. Tuck your shirt in.

Always look like a professional and act like one. Branding is everything.

85. Timing is everything.

Be on time, no matter what, even if they are not.

86. Accessorize with less.

No phones, coffee cups, TV or people watching.

87. Accountability is the key to cash.

Enforce payment, session and scheduling policies.

88. Obey the "One Way" rule.

Trainers are paid to listen not share personal information.

89. Sleeping with the Enemy.

Absolutely no sexual relationships with clients. The "Well" will go dry.

90. Keep your hand on the pulse.

Always monitor heart rates during workout sessions.

91. Respect the "All or Nothing" rule.

Educate and motivate clients on all components of wellness, do not piece meal your sessions with just weights.

92. Follow up for cash.

Never allow 48 hours between connecting with a current client. This helps client retention.

93. Never be afraid to say, "No."

If you don't know an answer to a question, say you don't; then within twenty-four hours get it.

94. Motivate by being methodical.

If possible do not go by a clock to stop your sessions. Be fluid, set a good pace and get as much accomplished as possible.

95. Enforce the "Technology Free" Zone.

Unless it's an emergency, do not allow phone calls, either by the client or you.

96. No shoes, no service.

Not only for safety sake, but to also to send a message on being serious, if they forget shoes, no session.

97. Ride the "Ten Week "wave and then get off.

If you have a set routine for a client change it up around the ten week mark. Anything more breeds stagnation.

98. Testing for Retention

Periodical fitness test around six to eight weeks better ensures your clients to stick with you.

99. Empty words equal empty wallets.

If at all possible, do not coach someone to do something that you are not willing to do or have done; these are words with out meaning to clients.

100. A joyful trainer is a RICH TRAINER.

What ever you do, enjoy your work, when you don't; it's time to do something else.

Conclusion

I would not take a million bucks for the *"On the Job or OJT,"* experience I have received over the last three decades. My classroom education got me started, but the real world taught me to keep going.

The fact is neither you nor I will learn everything there is to know; each day will be a new learning experience. What I have discovered is, you will definitely learn about yourself and what you're made of. OJT will mold you, define you and educate you on the REAL world.

Fitness Training is a people business more so than a numbers game. It requires more emotions and creativity than logic or reason; understand this and you will be RICH, neglect it and stay POOR.

Remember it's the little things that matter most in costumer care, at the same time it's the big picture that's most important when taking care of your business.

Never lose your Joy while in the trenches. No matter how dirty it may get, lose your reasons and lose your soul. Be a trainer to empower and inspire not for finances or fame; true intentions builds longevity.

There are mainly four things that separate RICH TRAINERS from POOR ones:

1. Sell outs!
2. ID's
3. Imaginations
4. Wolf Spiders

Treat being a fitness trainer from the beginning as a profession. It is a business, act like it is. Leave your EGO at the door, always; it will cost you the most money in the end. Your biggest competitor is not the trainer down the street; it's your lack of creativity in your head; avoid the competitive and nurture the creative. And never eat your own. Disrespecting, undercutting, bad mouthing fellow trainers only hurts the profession and your reputation more than anything else.

BONUS MATERIAL- RICH TRAINER Series

Here is a little bonus material; an excerpt from the Business 101 Part of the RICH TRAINER series.

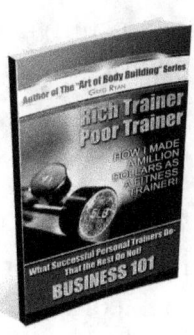

The "Gate Keepers"

You are only as good those around you. My father would preach this to me all the time. He always seemed to have good quality friends and business associates circling around.

Meet the Fockers; what a great movie. Jack (Robert De Niro), the gate keeper was always giving Greg (Ben Stiller) the business about, <u>"The Circle of Trust."</u> Or in other words; a small family like society of people who had your back no matter what. While earned, once in you never would have to leave; unless you royally screwed up.

The business centers on cultivating relationships; clients, associates or your inner circle and Gate Keepers.

Your Circle of Trust

I always seem to like team sports. Just watching a group of people come together for one common goal, fight off adversity, or just play for the love of the game was inspiring.
It didn't matter as much about the outcome as it did of what you learned about you and your team mates. You really are only as good at what you do as those you surround yourself with. You learned a lot about trust.

The Gate Keepers

Over the years I took my fathers advice and built a group of team players around me and my business; who I call, *"The Gate Keepers."* These individuals possess better than average business knowledge and practice as well as wonderful personal character. Gender, background or race matter not, it was about good sound business and life principles.

The Mission

The Mission or goal of the so called, *Gate Keepers* is what? One, what ever your business mission statement is. By the way, if you are serious about this RICH TRAINER thing, the first thing you should do is create a mission statement for your business.

Quality Not Quantity

The number of Gate Keepers is irrelevant, the type of people is most important. As you will see, I have a diverse group that fits all my business needs. You could have a few or many as long as the goal of the Gate Keeper philosophy is met.

-Trustworthy

A gate keeper had to be trustworthy first and foremost. I needed to count on them and not worry about things going on behind my back. Trust, not always an easy thing to read in people, is it?

-Loyal

A gate keeper had to be loyal. I did not want someone on my side one day and then flip to someone else another.

-Bold

Gate keepers had to have a spine. They must be bold in their beliefs and convictions; committed to the cause.

-Straight Shooters

I don't like fluff; just give it to me straight. I respect that out of another as well. Gate Keepers have to be straight shooters in my circle.

The Key Holders

For me I had a game plan of who I wanted guarding my gate. It would consist of people who specialized in important areas of my business. Such as......

Mentor

From start to finish you need a mentor. A mentor is a coach, counselor or teacher who you respect and look up to for advice. Don't abuse your relationship with to frequent of visits, but on a consistent basis, meet with a person you would consider a mentor. Everyone needs a mentor.

Accountability Partner

An accountability partner (AP) is a person who holds you to your goals and mission of your company. You meet on a regular basis, more so than a mentor. An AP is not a mentor and a mentor is not an AP. Whether you know it or not you get off track at times and need a friendly GPS to get you back on track.

CPA

Goes with out saying, but you need a trustworthy CPA who knows your business.

Financial Planner

A financial planner is different than a CPA.
A financial planner helps you with strategic planning of monies in the future. It should go along with your mission statement of your company.

No Family Members

A good rule of thumb is to not have family members as Gate Keepers. Family and business in ninety-five percent of the time do not mix. What starts out as good intentions; ends in wedges splitting the best of families apart; sometimes for good?

Who every you get to guard you gates, remember it's about quality not quantity. Gate Keepers can be the difference between freedom and poverty as a fitness trainer.

The Law of the Few

Some people call it the eighty-twenty rule. I like the way Malcolm Gladwell explains it in his book, <u>The Tipping Point.</u> He calls it, *"The Law of the Few."*

With the Oprah Winfrey attitude of structuring an empire and my fathers, "Gate Keeper" mentality of protecting the fort, I developed my own business template or philosophy to fit the fitness business. **Long term I wanted to create a system that I could duplicate anywhere at anytime.**

A *"Business Template"* is a certain way you choose to conduct your business; a mold, manual or guide, so to speak. My philosophy has always been simple,

Work smart and develop quality relationships with people, organizations and companies; spending as little on outside advertisement as possible.

In other words, create a group or network around you that works with and for your business 24/7. A *Network* is any netlike system that connects things, objects or people together.

The Law of a Few

The Oprah approach and the gate keepers are only as good for your business as the quality of people they allow *through*.

Growing up on a farm we sold our produce to a local market who distributed fruit and vegetables all over the country. In the beginning we had to go there to sell our crops. Over time my father developed meaningful relationships with selected buyers on the market. He would go for hours, even if he had nothing to sell, just to mingle with the buyers. He knew the importance of cultivating and nurturing not only his crops, but relationships as well. I just didn't seem to have his personality.

Interesting enough he only spent time with a selected few; they were sought out every time he perused the market. At the time, I never understood why he did so.

Over time, during the crop harvesting period we would get constant calls from mostly the, "selected few," buyers; each one placing substantial orders for our produce. For as long as I can remember, that few quality individuals supplied us all the orders we could handle without leaving our farm.

Malcolm Gladwell explains, <u>The Law of the Few,</u> like this,

"The majority of the work will be done by a handful of exceptional people who have the appropriate skill sets."

He goes onto say, there are three key types of people in the majority, connectors, mavens and salesman; each having a different role to play.

While challenging to find specifically one of each type or person, my goal at the time; **find a "few" quality people, organizations or companies to send me clients, and have them come to me when at all possible.** If a connector, one who was good at networking, a maven, up-to-date information geek and a salesman good at persuasion happened to be in the fold, then that was icing on the cake.

Observing my father convinced me that if I even only had a few good ones that, they could and would supply me with as much business as I would ever need. Looking back my father also taught me the smart way to fish.

The Best Fishing Hole

First, you spend time finding a great hole to fish out of; when you find it, stay there until you feel you've caught all the keepers. In other words, ask yourself,

"Who and what organization, company and profession have the same similar customer, client or patient base I want?" What professions are the fertile ponds and who in those professions are the biggest fish?

Here are the professions (ponds) I caught the biggest fish out of:

Orthopedic Surgeons
Physical Therapist/Occupational Therapist
Psychologist
Nutritionists
Endocrinologist
Spas

Fitness trainers make the mistake of not going back to the same pond or lake like gyms thinking clients are just going to appear. The gym has been all fished out.

So the first part of a good fitness training business template is to build a group of quality like minded professionals that you can network with. **This group if nurtured and developed can and will send you all the clients you will need, and guess what? FOR FREE!**

A word of caution, make sure they share the same philosophy and similar goals for their clients/customers you do. This is very important for your long term success; more than you will ever know.

Create a Win-Win

The best posturing you can have when you approach someone is to create a win-win relationship. With out making it noticeable, emphasize what you and your business can and will do to enhance their patients, customers, organizations or institutions.

Home Field Advantage

In any negotiating or sports event for that matter, you will have an advantage if it's on your own turf; you know the terrain. The second part of developing your template is to get them to come to you. This has many unseen benefits to you and your company; from scheduling, perceived value, comfort, confidence and retention. This is one area, where having your own facility is a big plus.

Referral Base Business

When people tell you that referrals are the cheapest way of getting new people through your door, they are not kidding. This type of business template has saved me more time, effort and money over the years than I can put a figure to. Nurture the relationships and the rest will follow.

Good luck and I hope you learn something.

Website: www.rich-trainer.com
Email: greg@resolutions.bz